"New Ideas For Gout Treatments with Gout remedies for Eliminating Uric Acid and Body Acids"

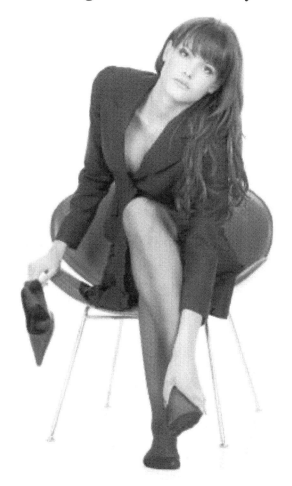

By Rudy S Silva, Natural Nutritionist

Table Of Contents

1: What Is This Gout Book All About?

It was thought at one time that gout was a disease that only the elderly, rich, and others who over ate developed this condition. However, with the increase in processed food and the appearance of junk food, those that favored this food became victims of an acid body and of excess uric acid.

The real cause of gout is an imbalance of the acid-alkaline balance in your body. There are two different types of acids that you need to be concerned with and eliminate when you have gout – acid body and uric acid.

How this acid-alkaline imbalance occurs, how it creates gout, and what you can do about it is what this book is all about.

Once you rebalance your acids, you not only get rid of gout, but you create an alkaline body that is less susceptible to disease.

Gout and Arthritis

Gout is expressed as form of arthritis, "gouty arthritis," muscle or tissue pain in your body, but is not arthritis. I'm sure many of you have had some form of pain in your legs or calves that woke you up, at night giving you agonizing pain, if you move your legs. Now, this might not be gout, but this is the type of pain that gout sufferers experience, but only more painful and mostly located in their joints.

If you have gout, you may experience piercing sharp pain in your joints, toes, ankles, knees, shoulders or elbows. This pain comes from the formation of needle-like uric crystals that precipitate and attach themselves to your cartilage, muscle tissue, skin tissue or synovial pouches in your joints. These uric crystals come from excess uric acid that travels throughout your blood, and which drops out of your blood to form crystals. Not all people with excess uric acid develop gout. But, if they do, there are other illnesses that they may develop, without knowing it.

Uric acid is not only responsible for gout, but is the seed for kidney stones.

In this book, you will get a complete understanding of what gout is and what is presently known about this condition. In addition, you will find out how to cure this condition, using the right foods, techniques, supplements, fruits, and remedies. You will also find out what drugs are presently used to treat gout.

What Causes Gout

Scientists, medical researchers, doctors, or alternative practitioners often say that they don't know what causes gout. But, there are plenty of evidence and information available from many studies that point to specific reasons for gout to form.

You will be given a good picture of what causes gout. From this information, you will be able to see how various natural remedies presented will help you cure or eliminate your gout.

Family History

First of all, studies have shown that if your family members suffer from gout, your chance of having gout are 20% higher. The reason for this might come from the way you developed you're eating habit, as a child. Most family members all eat the same food and may develop unhealthy eating habits. The impact of poor eating habits will be discussed in later chapters. Heredity is also a factor for family members to develop a tendency toward high uric acid levels. When this occurs, more attention by these family members needs to be made on diet.

Your Medical conditions

There are various medical conditions that can increase your risk of developing gout. When you have an illness and or are taking drugs, this situation means that you have an acid body. When you have an acid body, you are more prone to having gout. Here are four conditions that contribute to gout.

1. high blood pressure (hypertension)
2. diabetes, both type 1 diabetes and type 2 diabetes
3. kidney disease
4. hypothyroidism
5. having high levels of fat and cholesterol levels in your blood

Kidney Disease

Your kidney is responsible for eliminating excess uric acid from your blood. In some people, the kidney may be diseased and not able to remove all the uric acid it needs to from the blood.

Hypothyroidism

Not all people with hypothyroidism have gout, but those with hypothyroidism tend to have high levels of uric acid. When these people are under hypothyroidism medication, this tends to control their gout.

Diabetics

People with diabetes tend to have higher levels of uric acid than normal. When people have an insulin resistance condition, this causes excess uric acid.

See A Doctor

There are many other body conditions or illnesses that may appear as gout. So, see your doctor, to confirm it is gout and not some other serious condition.

2: What Is The Real Truth About Gout?

Gout is an inflammatory disease. When inflammation occurs anywhere in your body, it occurs because something is irritating, burning, or damaging your body's tissues.

Gout is an inflammation of various bone joints and is considered a form of arthritis. This inflammation occurs when **monosodium urate monohydrate crystals** deposit or precipitate in your joints or in the joint synovial fluid. When these crystals form, they contain sharp points, which tear or cut into cartilage, bone ligaments, and tissue, causing great pain and discomfort.

These crystals can also deposit in major organs, causing major damage. For this reason, it's important to take action on this disease to eliminate it and stop its return.

This gout pain often comes at night, when you are deep asleep. The sharp pains appear in your toes, joints or calves. Any movement of your legs increases the pain. The pain can be unbearable at times.

Gout pain may last for days or even weeks, and the time between attacks can be weeks or years.

Pesudogout

There is pesudogout that mimics the conditions of gout, but this occurs when calcium pyrophosphate crystals collect in various joints causing pain and inflammation, like in a typical gout condition.

Pesudogout is not caused by high levels of uric acid, but is an imbalance of minerals that keeps calcium out of solution.

When you don't have enough of the mineral sodium in your body, calcium will precipitate into crystals called bone spurs. This condition will also be eliminated with the information in this book.

What Causes Urate Crystals to Form?

Urate crystals form when you have an imbalance in your acid-alkaline levels. When you have an excess of acid in your body, uric acid will tend to precipitate and form crystals.

So, if you have an alkaline body, you will not have gout. If you have an acid body, your chances of having gout are higher.
To get rid of gout you will find in later chapters many ways to make your body more alkaline.

Purine is Uric Acid

Gout also occurs when an excess of meat or other food, which contain a high level of purines is eaten.

So, what are purines? Purines occur in all foods and plants. They help to form the chemical structure of genes. When you eat food, the genes in this food are broken down, during digestion and purine is released. This purine is now uric acid. It remains in the blood, dissolved and harmless.

When your old cells die and decomposed, purine is released into your blood. This is another source of uric acid.

Typically, 70% of the urate produced daily is eliminated by your kidneys in urine. The other 30% is routed to your liver and moved into your gallbladder and into your colon, where it is removed by your stools.

When too much purine food is eaten and uric acid is produced, hyperuricaemia, by your body, your body has to figure out how to get rid of it.

Too much uric acid can also remain in your body, if your kidneys are not functioning properly. Your kidneys will not remove the 70%. If your liver doesn't remove the 30% it is required to, excess uric acid can remain in your blood.

The Insulin Factor

When an excess of insulin is formed, by eating an excess of carbohydrates or when your cells become insulin resistant, an excess of urate can be created, leading to a buildup of uric acid in your blood.

If you are obesity, have type 2 diabetes, high blood pressure, or have a kidney disease, you are more susceptible to increases in uric acid levels.

The Forming of Urate Crystals

Gout is formed when the urate concentration in your blood becomes super saturated and precipitates, forming monosodium urate crystals in various joints and sometimes in tissue.

When crystals form within joints, they can come loose and redeposit in synovial sacs and cause chronic inflammatory arthritis.

Kidney stones can also develop from excess urate, when the urate precipitates within the kidney. Specific research has uncovered that certain variant genes are associated with reduced ability of the kidney to excrete uric acid.

Other Gout Causes

In some cases, gout is caused by heredity, eating habits, and environmental exposures.

Gout or increases in blood uric acid can also be caused by excess molybdenum. If you work in milling, paints, mining, lubricants, fertilizers or armor plating, these jobs or areas are high in molybdenum.

Gout Attacks

Gout attacks occur for a short time, but are quite painful, when they occur. In some cases, a gout attack can happen on occasion or frequently. When gout attacks occur frequently or take some time to disappear, these attacks can cause weakening, deformation, or destruction of your joints.

How Does Uric Acid Buildup In Your Blood?

In normal people, the amount of uric acid that is created from daily eating, body exercise, or cell activities is expelled from the body, and no gout is ever experienced. However, in some people,

1. Uric acid, which is created from the breakdown of old cells, and the construction of new one is not removed fast enough by the kidneys, builds up in the blood

2. Their kidneys do not eliminate enough uric acid and the uric blood level rises

3. They over exercise causing an excess of uric acid to build up in their blood

4. They become dehydrated, by not drinking plenty of water, during the day or during strenuous exercise. Less liquid in your body cause uric acid to rise. More frequent urination reduces the uric acid in your blood

5. They become ill or come down with more infections than normal, causing more uric acid in their blood

6. They have hypothyroidism, leukemia, psoriasis, or lymphoma

7. They injured a joint creating a weak point where uric acid crystals can deposit easily

8. They start to lose weight too fast, using various diet programs, which interrupt the excretion of uric acid through their urine

9. Their overweight condition leads to an increase chance of a gout attack. Extra pounds cause the body to produce more uric acid and also to block the excretion of this uric acid from the body

10. They have excess stress or are extra nervous, which cause uric acid to rise in the blood

11. They drink up to a dozen cans of beer or 2 ½ liters. Alcohol slows down the excretion of uric acid in the kidneys

12. They drink an excess of sodas, which contain sugar or fructose and this causes uric acid

13. They have a previous joint injury

14. They use recreational drugs or medical drugs for other diseases

15. They have a tumor

16. They have lead poisoning

17. They have a digestive enzyme deficiency causing poor digestion and excess acid waste in the stomach

3: Medical Treatments Used For Gout

Gout can be treated effectively with diet and natural remedies. Most doctors will not tell you this. But, if you wish to use medical treatment for your gout, here is what you can expect.

Gout Attack

The recommended treatment for a gout attack is the use NSAIDs or Non-steroidal Anti-inflammatory Drugs, such as naproxen, 500mg for every 10 hours.

If you can't tolerate NSAIDs, then corticosteroids are recommended. If you don't like corticosteroids, then colchicine is the drug to take.

Drugs for Gout

There are some medicines, which can reduce your risk of future gout attacks. These are usually taken after an attack is over.

Nonsteroidal Anti-Inflammatories (NSAIDs) - Indocin, Indomethicin, Ibuprofen, Naproxen, Naprosyn, Aleve – These drugs decrease gout inflammation and pain. Their side effects are nausea, abdominal pain or bleeding, indigestion, dizziness, and stomach ulcers.

Allopurinol (Ayloprim) is currently the most widely used medicine to reduce urate levels. It blocks the enzymatic conversion of hypoxanthine and xanthine to urate.

Benzbromarone is used when allopurinol has failed to lower serum urate concentrations. It is a uricosuric medicine that increases the net renal excretion rate of urate – urine.

Benzbromarone inhibits the action of urate transporters in the renal tubules, leading to increased renal excretion of urate – urine.

Probenecid (Benemid, Probalan) Anturance is used to reduce the amount of uric acid in your body by simulating the kidneys for increase urine output. Some side effects are intestinal irritation, stomach aches, and skin rashs.

Colchincine inhibits inflammation and decreases joint pain. Side effects are diarrhea.

Corticosteroids are anti-inflammatory hormones, which are taken orally or injected into the affected area. The side effects include a decrease immune function and bone thinning.

febuxostat (Uloric) is a xanthine oxidase inhibitor that works by decreasing the amount of uric acid made in the body. This drug must be used daily. It usually takes months before this drug starts to prevent gout attacks. The side effects are liver damage.

Pegloticase (Krystexxa) converts uric acid to allantoin, which remains in the blood better than uric acid. This drug is given every two weeks by intravenous infusion. Side effects are Nausea, vomiting and allergic reactions.

There are also some drugstore products that you can use for gout. These include diuretics to produce more urine and aspirin to reduce pain. Using diuretics removes water from your body, but blocks the removal of uric acid, whereas, aspirin can increase your uric acid levels.

4: Foods That Create Gout Acids

There are some doctors who say diet does not affect gout. This is often said about various diseases, but this can't be true, since you are what you eat. Eating a lot acid food, keeps your blood and lymph liquid acidic. This in turn increases the possibility of uric acid precipitating into harmful crystals. It also favors a variety of other diseases.

Certain foods can activate a gout attack, in your joints and especially in your feet, ankles and legs. Eating excess purine foods has been identified as the chemical that leads to gout. But, other unbalanced body conditions contribute also to gout. Not all people with excess uric acid in their blood form or create urate crystals. And, uric acid is not only created by food, but your body also creates it, when dead cells are broken down. There many other ways uric acid is created in your body.

Fats or fatty foods also play an important part in gout. If you have a diet high in fats, these fats prevent your kidneys from removing the amount of uric acid that it should. The result is that an excess of uric acid remains in your blood.

Now, even though you might have high uric acid in your blood and don't form gout, it does not mean that you are healthy. High uric acid in your blood is a condition you don't want, since it leads to many other diseases.

But, covered in this chapter are the foods that are high in purine, and that you should cut back on, if you are prone to gout attacks. You don't have to eliminate these foods from your diet forever. In fact, you may just need to limit the amount that you eat.

After you complete this program, you will find that you will not need to cut back, because you may be using many of the diet changes listed here. The diet in this program helps you create an alkaline body, which makes you less susceptible to gout.

Meat

All animal meat contains purine, such as red meat, organ meat, meat extracts, and some fish. So cut back on these meats.

Some of the fish to avoid are herring, sardines, and mussels.

Alcohol

Beer has always been suggested to avoid, when you have gout. But, it is also best to eliminate all alcohol beverages, when you are in a gout attack.

Baked Goods

Baked goods, which have yeast, also contain purines and should be avoided.

Soft Drinks

Soft drinks and other sugary drinks, which are high in fructose, can cause an excess of uric acid in your blood. Just one or two drinks a day can cause you uric acid problems. Fruit juices can also cause uric problems, if they are not fresh and don't have enough fiber in them.

Body Illnesses

Certain illnesses such as severe psoriasis or blood disorders create an excess of uric acid. If you have high blood pressure, kidney damage, obesity, diabetes, and many other diseases, you will be more susceptible to gout.

Gout can also be associated with physical injuries, surgery, long hospitalization, or using drugs.

Gout may also show up, when you have some cancers or tumors.

Gout is not always just a symptom that comes for a short time. Many people experience gout for weeks and sometimes for extended periods.

Conditions That Create Gout

- Obesity
- Heavy alcohol consumption
- Diets high in purine foods, seafood, meat, meat organs
- Extremely low-calorie diets
- Always using aspirin
- Regular use of niacin
- Frequently drinking high-fructose drinks
- Quick weight loss
- Kidney disease
- High blood pressure
- Psoriasis
- Tumors
- Hemolytic anemia
- Lead poisoning
- Hypothyroidism Surgery

Foods to avoid, if you have gout

Here is a list of food that you need to minimize or eliminate from your diet.

- Avoid or minimize the use Scallops, herring, tuna, anchovies and meat during a gout attack.
- Reduce the use of red meat, chicken, pork, turkey or lamb
- Avoid eating animal skin and fatty meat.
- Limit the use of bouillon, commercially prepared gravies or soups.
- Limit your use of chocolates
- Avoid sodas and sugar, corn syrup, or fructose sweetened drinks
- Avoid sweetbreads, chips, sugary products, and junk food
- Avoid or minimize the use asparagus, cauliflower, spinach, and mushrooms, peas, beans and legumes
- Eliminate completely liver and kidney meat
- Stop drinking Beer tea, coffee, cocoa
- Minimize your use of oats, but you can use them occasionally

5: Foods That Stop Gout Pain

There are many foods that you can eat to help you clear your gout. For gout pain that occurs for 15 to 30 minutes a day or more, apply the principles listed in the chapters on burning acid and body cycles. These practices will eliminate and cure your infrequent gout attacks. In addition, these practices are the foundation of creating a healthy body.

If you have gout attacks that remain for days, then you need to follow the food practices, in the previous chapter, that will not aggravate your gout.

Increase your consumption of vegetables and fruits in all forms. When you do this, you are helping your body excrete purine chemicals from your body and create an alkaline body. Your basic diet should be a moderate protein and fat intake, with no internal organs.

Dairy products are good to eat such as,

- Milk and non-fermented milk products
- Eggs whites, hard boiled for the egg whites
- Cottage cheese, mozzarella cheese
- Whey protein
- Shrimp, lobster, eel, and crab in moderation.
- Complex carbohydrates, brown rice, wheat bread, pasta
- Citrus fruits, non-sweeten juices
- Herbal teas, Coffee
- Water

Egg whites, milk, and whey protein do not have purines, and

this is why they are on the list of foods to eat. However, yogurt and aged cheeses are not on the eat list.

Eating low-fat dairy is recommended for gout. Use skim milk or low-fat yogurt.

Water

Drinking plenty of water is necessary, to clear your gout. This increases the frequency of urination, and when you urinate, your kidneys excrete uric acid from your blood.

Purines in Food

Purines cannot be entirely avoided, because they occur in produce and other foods. In addition, they are created in your body as a result of recycling dead cells.

Apple

Eat at least two apples per day to neutralize uric acid. Eat them between meals and not after a meal. Apples will also give you relief from gout pain and reduce its inflammation.

Apple and Carrots

Eating carrots and apples is a great way to reduce gout acid and pain. One way to get daily relief is to juice apples and carrots together. Make a mixture of 1:1, or make 3/4 apple juice with 1/4 carrot juice.

Use carrots in any way that you can, either raw or cooked. The more carrots you eat the fewer issues you will have with gout.

Avocados

Avocados are high in essential fatty acids that help to reduce body pain.

Celery

It is recommended that you take a supplement of celery seeds, when you have gout. While waiting to get the seeds, you can eat 4-5 celery sticks per day with the leaves. This will help you to lower your uric blood levels.

Juice of Cucumber, Carrot, Spinach

A juicer is a great tool to have. You can create all kinds of juices, when you have to. Creating a juice of cucumber, carrots and spinach can help you get rid of a lot of uric acid. Cucumber is a strong diuretic and will help to produce more urine.

Add some apple to this cucumber mixture, to sweeten up this juice. Then, you will be able to drink more of it.

Artichoke

When you eat artichokes, they have the ability to reduce the production of uric acid, in your body. Not all people like artichokes and you have to develop a taste for them.
Artichokes have excellent health benefits, such as body detoxifying, cholesterol lowering, and liver repair.

Bananas

Bananas can treat gout. They are high in potassium and other minerals, which convert uric crystals into liquid. Eat only two to three bananas per day. Choose those bananas that are not over ripe, but just right for eating.

Red or Black Cherries or Strawberries

Tart Cherries contain anti-inflammatory and potent antioxidants chemicals, such as flavonols and the Anthocyanins, which is an anti-inflammatory antioxidant.

This is a well-known remedy for gout, but researchers have found it hard to discover why cherries relieve gout. Despite many stories about how people were helped with gout by drinking or eating cherries, there are still some people that are not helped. If cherries don't reduce your gout symptoms, then move on to eating other foods that do.

In a well-documented story, 1950, Ludwig Blau, Ph.D. reported in the *Texas Reports on Biology and Medicine* that he cured his gout that had him in a wheel chair. He did this by eating or drinking cherries every day. He found that as long as he ate cherries, he had no gout pain. He used 6–8 cherries per day.

More cherries can be eaten, but 6 to 8 are the minimum. You can also use cherry extract, to prepare a cherry drink or to add to a fruit smoothie.

Fresh cherries always work best for gout, since the nutrients are in higher concentration. But frozen ones also work.

Pineapples and Juice

Eat pineapples and pineapple juice to ease your joint pain. Pineapples, with the protein digestive enzyme bromelain, help to reduce joint inflammation.

Grapes

Grapes are high in minerals that move your body toward alkalinity. Any slight movement towards an alkaline body means less uric acid will form uric crystals.

This little fruit will reduce the acidity of uric acid and then helps to eliminate it through your kidneys.

Nuts

Eat a variety of nuts, but do it in moderation.

Fish

You need to eat some type of fish. It has been found that fish oil provides lubricant to your joints. Without some form of lubricant, your joints will wear down your cartilage as they rub together. You can supplement with a good fish oil capsule, to provide this lubricant.

Seaweed

All seaweed is beneficial in curing gout. These foods contain a high level of minerals. The balance of these minerals is in a way that your body needs them. They will make your body more alkaline, because of the calcium, potassium, and sodium they contain.

Vegetables and Fruits

Concentrate on vegetables, like sweet potatoes, squashes, cabbage, and potatoes. You can prepare them any way you like. Also, eat many of the other vegetables you like.

Both vegetables and fruits are high in antioxidants and minerals. Antioxidants help fight off damage to your joints and reduce inflammation. Minerals make your body less acidic and keep uric acid in solution and not in crystal form.

Vegetable Juices

If you have a juicer, then you are prepared to fight various diseases. By creating the juice of a combination of vegetables, you can produce a high alkaline drink that will keep your gout away.

Dandelion Leaves - Vegetable Salads

When you make a green salad, add some dandelion, kale, and spinach leaves. All the salad leaves are high in minerals and help make your body more alkaline.

Gout Diet

6: Curing Gout With Natural Remedies

Creating Uric Acid

Losing weight leads to substances the stop the excretion of your uric acid. Keeping your weight or losing it at a slower rate can help reduce gout attacks. Don't eat less the 1700 1900 calories per day, but this just a guide line.

It has been found that one of the best approaches for eliminating gout or for controlling it is to move your body from an acid state to an alkaline state. This is done by concentrating on foods that produce an alkaline residue, when your cells metabolize nutrients. You can increase your transition from acid to alkaline, by taking alkaline minerals with your meals.

Here some of the most effective natural remedies that have been used to minimize or eliminate gout pain.

Alfalfa

Alfalfa is packed with minerals, which will make your body more alkaline. This is one of the things that will help you cure your gout. You can take it in capsule form or in powder. There are many green drinks that contain alfalfa, and many other green grasses that make an excellent morning drink for your gout.

Apple Cider Vinegar

Apple cider vinegar has been found to work for many ailments. For gout, here's what you need to do.

Take 2 teaspoons of organic apple cider vinegar and add 2

teaspoons of honey. Do these two times a day. This remedy will reduce your gout pain, within a few hours.

You can mix 1 to 2 tablespoon of apple cider vinegar in 8 oz. of water and drink it, once per day. You can add a bit of honey, if you need to.

Baking Soda

Baking soda helps to lower the amount of uric acid in your blood. When you do this, you will get relief from joint pain. Here's how to use it.

Place 1/2 teaspoon of baking soda in 8 oz of water and drink it. You can do this three times a day only. If you have high blood pressure, **don't use this remedy.**

Limit your use of this remedy, since it will change the pH of your stomach acid.

Celery Seed

Here is another remedy that is great for gout pain. You can eat one tablespoon of celery seeds per day, or you can take celery seed capsules. Celery seeds have the compound "Sedanolide," which is used in other herbal remedies for gout inflammation.

Dandelion Extract

Dandelion extract is useful for gout, since it contains a lot of **Potassium**. This mineral can neutralize body acids and reduce your body acid load, making your body more alkaline. When this happens, uric acid is more likely to remain in solution, instead of precipitating into damaging crystal deposits.

If you can't get dandelion extract, try getting the herb and making a tea. Allow the herb to sit in hot water for 10 to 15 minutes to make it stronger. Add some honey to give it more flavor.

Devil's Claw

Devil's claw will provide you anti-inflammatory benefits and lower uric acid levels, which can help with your gout pain.
If you have diabetes or are taking a blood-thinning drug **do not take this herb**.

Boswellia

Boswellia is an Indian herb that has shown to control arthritis. It reduces inflammation and promotes circulation in the affected areas. It is good for gout inflammation.

Drinking Water

Drinking a lot of water, when you have gout is a smart idea. Uric acid is removed by your kidneys through your urine. The more you urinate the less uric acid you have in your body. The more uric acid you have in your body the more likely you will form uric acid crystals in your joints.

So, drink 6 – 7 glasses of water per day. If you eat fruits and fruit juices without sugar or fructose, you can count this as water also. Herbal teas can also be counted as water, but not regular tea.

Ice Water

Using an ice pack on your gout inflammation can quickly reduce your pain. Use this idea with other remedies listed here. An ice pack will only provide temporary relief.

You can also make an ice bath, which is not fully loaded with ice, but just enough to create a cold bath that will remove some of the pain and burning joint sensation. Use this bath until it starts to reach room temperature.

Epsom Salt

A warm foot bath with Epsom salt is another good gout remedy. In a foot tub, add warm water and 1/2 cup of Epsom salt. If you need more salt, add a slight more. Soak your foot or feet, until the water gets cold. Do this once a week. You will be absorbing many of the minerals in the Epsom salt, which will make your body more alkaline.

Garlic

Garlic should be used in all cooking and taken in supplements, because of its long list of health benefits it provides. For gout, it has been shown to reduce joint pain and gout symptoms.

Ginger Root

Ginger root has anti-inflammatory properties. Here's how to use it.

1. Drink a glass of ginger root tea every day.

2. Use ginger root in your cooking every day.

3. Create a paste of ginger root and apply it to the affected area.

4. Ground 1/3 cup of ginger and place it in a foot tub of warm water. Soak your affected foot for 30 minutes. This will help to eliminate some of your uric acid. Rinse your foot off with water, after your 30 minutes.

Green Powder or Capsules

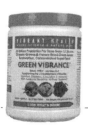

A good green called **Green Vibrance** provides you with a variety of green grasses. It's these grasses that contain the minerals and other nutrients that you need to eliminate gout.

Green Vibrance contains organic barley, oat, wheat, Kamut, alfalfa sprouts, broccoli sprouts, spirulina, chlorella, rice bran, and many more vegetables.

Grape seed or pine bark extracts.

These extracts are high in antioxidants and will neutralize damaging free radicals, in your joints and tissue. They work as an anti-inflammatory remedy. You can put this extract over the affected joint.

Juniper Oil

Place a compress of juniper oil on your affected area. Juniper oil will help to break down the uric crystals.

Placing this on the affected area will help break down the toxic deposits.

Lemon Juice

Lemon juice is a powerful remedy for gout. Even though its juice is acidic, when this juice is metabolized at the cell level, it creates what is called an alkaline ash or residue, which will neutralize acid. This makes your body more alkaline, and your uric acid tends to remains as liquid, when your body is more alkaline.

First, when you first wake up, drink 8 oz. of distilled water with the juice of one lemon and do this three times per day. Add a little honey to sweeten this drink, if you like.

Here's another way to use lemon. Juice one lemon and add it to 1/2 teaspoon of baking soda. Mix these ingredients, and then add it to 8 oz. of water. Then, drink up.

Milk Thistle

Milk Thistle is known as a liver tonic and can protect the liver from toxins, as found in gout medications. You need a healthy liver, so it can move uric acid out through your gallbladder and colon.

Ruby Reds

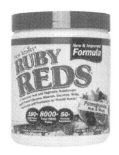

Ruby Reds is a powder supplement that contains over 50 natural ingredients of fruits, vegetables, fiber, probiotics and digestive enzymes. This is an excellent powder that you can add to your smoothies or to create a morning drink with juice. This supplement gives you an excellent source of antioxidants and minerals that will help you with your gout. This is a Delicious Fruit and Vegetable Supplement with the right vitamins, minerals, enzymes, herbs, nutrients and probiotics for overall health. One glass gives you the antioxidant power of 13 servings of fruits and vegetables.

Rutin

Rutin is good for reducing gout inflammation. It also reduces uric acid and prevents it from forming joint crystals.

You can buy rutin as a supplement, which is a nice way to get it.

Willow Bark

Willow contains compounds as salicylates from which aspirin is created. Using a strong tea of willow can help you relieve pain and inflammation.

Yucca Herb Stock Leaf

Yucca Herb has antioxidants, anti-inflammatory, free-radical scavenging, anti-arthritic properties, and anti-inflammatory benefits. Drink this every day, for gout.

Turmeric Root

Turmeric has benefits for arthritis because of its anti-inflammatory properties and thus helps reduce gout pain. It does this by the curcumin that it has, which blocks prostaglandins that produce pain in your body. This chemical process is similar to the action of aspirin and ibuprofen, but not as strong.

You can take turmeric root in capsules to get a high dose. Or you add a curry dish to your weekly diet.

Other Natural Gout Treatments

Magnets

Magnets have been used for gout, since Cleopatra during the Roman Empire. This type of application is not to be taken lightly, since magnets have been use by many, for body pain.
A magnet of 950 gauss is typically applied to the blood vessels near the pain. Relief is felt within minutes. Place a magnet inside your sock and one on the outside of your sock to keep the one inside in place. You can keep it in place, for as long as you want.

7: Supplements and Remedies That Cure Gout

There is one supplement that you need to avoid, niacin. This supplement can create a gout attack, since the nicotinic acid it creates in your blood competes with uric acid in your kidneys to be excreted. If you are using niacin under a doctor's care for cardiovascular conditions, check with your doctor about eliminating it, if you have gout.

There are not very many supplements to take for gout. But, of the few that are, vitamin C is one that you should be taking. Vitamin C is used by your body for a variety of different body conditions, so you should be taking it, even though you may not have gout.

Vitamin C supplements

In a 2009 vitamin C study, vitamin C showed a reduced risk of developing gout. This study had 46,994 men who were followed for several years. It compared men with a vitamin C intake of less than 250 mg a day. The result was that those men whose vitamin C intake of 1,000-1,499 mg per day had a 34% lower risk of gout.

And, for those men who took 1,500+ mg per day, they had a 45% lower risk of gout.

Taking vitamin C for gout makes a lot sense. It appears that vitamin C works by reducing the uric acid in your blood. It may do this by excreting more of it out your urine than normal.

Folic Acid

Folic acid is used in your body in the breakdown of proteins.

It also blocks the action of an enzyme that is responsible for forming uric acid.

You should use from 200 to 400 micrograms per day.

No side effects have been reported, when taking high doses of folic acid. Folic acid in these high doses has been shown to be as effective as the drug allopurinol.

High doses of folic acid should be taken with a doctor's care, since they can mask the deficiency of vitamin B12.

Alpha Lipoic Acid

There are chemicals called leukotrienes, which are involved in joint inflammation. You can reduce this inflammation by taking alpha lipoic acid with vitamin E and selenium. Here's the dose to take:

Alpha lipoic Acid, 50 to 800 mg per day

Vitamin E, 200 to 400 IU per day

Selenium, 200 micrograms per day

Bromelain

Bromelain is a digestive enzyme found in pineapple and is an effective anti-inflammatory.

Take Bromelain, 500 to 1,500 GDUs (Gelatin digestion units)

Essential fatty Acids

The essential fatty acids, omega-3, omega-6, and omega-9 are anti-inflammatory substances. You can get them in a variety of sources, such as fish oil, flax seed oil, evening primrose, olive oil, and other oils. It is best to use fish oil for gout.
Use Fish oil, 1,200 to 2,000 mg per day

Fruits

Lemon is also a very rich source of vitamin C, which helps in dissolving the gouty deposits. This is one of the efficient natural remedies for gout.

Increase the intake of citrus fruits, berries, tomatoes, green pepper and leafy green vegetables, which have a high content of vitamin C. They reduce inflammation produced in gouts. The amalaki (Indian Gooseberry) is one of the richest sources of vitamin C.

Make it a point to eat about three to four fresh fruits every day. This is one of the best diets for gout.

Seeds

Use both celery and kelp seed capsules. These seed capsules are high in minerals that can help neutralize your body acids and make you more alkaline.

8: Check Your Gout Level With pH Testing

Here is a way to do your own acid testing to see how acidic your body is. You want your body to be slightly alkaline so that you can get rid of gout and not have it return. You will not have gout, when your body is in an alkaline condition. When your body favors an alkaline condition, your uric acid tends to stay in liquid form and does not precipitate into crystals.

In this chapter and the next, you will discover one of the secrets of being healthy. Most people have an acid body, and this is why they come down with a variety of illnesses, including gout. Improve your acid-alkaline balance to where your body is slightly alkaline, and you will not only eliminate gout for good, but gain great health benefits.

You will be doing both a saliva and urine pH, but you will be starting with the saliva tests.

Here are 3 simple tests that you can do with your pH paper. These tests give you an idea of how alkaline your body is and how strong your alkaline reserves are. Knowing this will tell you how acidic your body is. The more acidic your body is the higher chance you have of having gout. Write down your readings and keep track of each test.

Saliva Test

Here is a simple test you can perform on your saliva that will give you an idea of where you stand, with your body's pH level. Your saliva contains mineral salts that keep it alkaline at 7.4. If your body is deficient in alkaline food or minerals, this test will show a pH lower than 7.4. The lower the drop in pH the less alkaline minerals you have in your body.

Keep in mind there are some inaccuracies with this method, since your body fluids are always in transition. This test simply gives you an idea of what your saliva pH is at that moment. Use this information for your own education. Then as you begin to change your eating habits and lifestyle, you can retest to see if there is a difference.

Three-Day pH Test

By testing your pH regularly, you can decide the validity of using pH litmus paper to determine the level of your health. As you make changes, you can test your saliva and urine to see if the pH litmus color changes.

You need to take this test for 3 days and at least 3 times a day and get an average value so that you can establish a base line or a starting point for yourself.

Here is a series of pH tests that you need to do that will determine what your health base line is. This will give you an indication of how acidic your body is, and how much you need to do to make it alkaline.

What to Expect from Your Saliva pH

Here is a simple test you can perform on your saliva that will give you an idea of where you stand with your body's pH level. Your saliva pH should be between 6.6 and 7.4, normal range.

If your saliva is below normal, you can influence your saliva's pH to read higher, by eating more acid binding (acid binding food will be explained in the next chapter) food and to supplement with potassium, magnesium and calcium.

Keep in mind there are some inaccuracies with this method, since your body fluids are always in transition. This test simply gives you an idea of what your saliva pH is, at that moment. Use this information for your own education. Then, as you begin to change your eating habits and lifestyle, you can retest to see, if there is a difference.

Starting Your Saliva Test

Gather saliva in your mouth then swallow. Do this two times. Place the pH paper under your tongue. Let it sit there for 5 seconds to wet it and then remove it. Let it sit for 20 seconds, compare the color of your pH paper to the color chart on the bottle and record the pH.

Do this test around one hour before eating or around two hours after eating. This reading gives you an idea about the state of your saliva. Your first test should be done first thing in the morning, before you rinse out your mouth or drink anything.

Saliva and Lemon Test

Now, do this test immediately after you do your morning saliva test.

- Squeeze half of lemon juice in one ounce of water, swish it around in your mouth for 5 seconds, and then spit it out.
- Now, wait one minute.
- Then, place the litmus paper into your mouth and wet it.
- Record your reading after one minute.
-

Now compare the color and pH value of this reading with your morning pH saliva reading. This reading should have a higher reading than your first saliva reading. For example,

- Morning reading is 6.5 pH (the higher the better)
- After the lemon test reading 6.9 pH
-

These readings are good, and indicate you have somebody mineral stores.

Now, suppose your readings were,

- First reading 6.5
- Lemon test reading 6.2

There is a drop in your lemon pH, and this is not too good. This means that you don't have enough minerals in your body to neutralize the acid in your mouth. You will have to eat more acid binding food.

Again, if your lemon test readings have a higher pH reading than your first reading, it means you have alkaline reserves. The bigger the difference between your first test and second test, the stronger your alkaline reserves. A small alkaline upward change means you have alkaline reserves, but they are not as strong as they should be.

If your lemon pH reading does not change from your first reading or actually goes down by becoming more acidic, then your alkaline reserves are weak, and you need to make some major changes in the way you eat. This also means you have a highly acidic body that can create some serious illness, especially if your lemon test pH is down to 6.0 and below.

Here is what your various saliva pH values mean.

The normal reading for saliva pH is 6.6 to 7.4.

pH level of 6.5 to 7.4 - You are at a **healthy level.** But, the higher number is better.

pH level of 6.0 to 6.5 – You may **not be feeling good and are starting to create disease.**

pH level of 5.0 to 6.0 - You have **major health problems.**

pH level of 4.5 – 5.0 – You **have a terminal disease.**

You are considered to have an alkaline body, if your overall body liquid is a pH of 6.5 to 7.4. The pH level you should strive for is 6.8 to 7.2. Higher pH values of 7.5 to 8.5 and up are also considered detrimental.

Urine pH test

The urine pH test and saliva test data needs to be combined to come up with an overall average pH reading. Only combine the first morning saliva pH and not the lemon pH reading with the urine pH.

There have been clinical studies, indicating that urine pH is an accurate reflection of your body responding to the production acid waste.

Each time you test your urine, note what you have eaten in your previous evening meal. Eating a high-protein meal, which is an acid meal, will require more body alkaline minerals to neutralize this dinner. If you eat a meal high in vegetables and little protein, then your body should easily neutralize the acid, from your meal by morning.

Here's how to do the urine pH test.

In the morning, when you urinate, allow it to flow for a couple of seconds, and then wet your pH litmus paper with urine.

pH Results

If your morning urine pH is below 6.4 and is more like 6.0 or below, this indicates that your body did not have enough alkaline minerals to neutralize your evening dinner. In addition, you do not have enough alkaline mineral reserves to protect your body from acid and toxic damage to your cells and tissues.

A urine good range is 5.8 to 6.5 If your urine is down to 5.8, this is on the low side, but is considered ok. But, this is not a good place for your pH to be at all the time. You want your urine pH to be close to 6.5. This shows that you have plenty of mineral stores to neutralize a previous night's acid dinner – meat or carbohydrates.

If your morning urine is over 7.5 to 8.0, this indicates your body is going into an emergency state, using ammonia from your liver in an effort to reduce your acid body. If you read as high as 8.0, for sure you are producing ammonia to neutralize your acid dinner. To change this will require a substantial change in your eating habits. Sometimes you can smell that your urine is ammonia like. Keep in mind that this may be temporary, but if you consistently see this pH value, then you definitely have a problem and need to back off from eating acid food.

Test your urine for three to four days, to see if it remains consistent. Record this information to see how it changes, as you progress through this program and change your eating habits.

- Measure your saliva pH in the morning.
- Measure your morning urine
- Measure your urine pH two times during the day.
- Measure your urine mid-day, two hours after eating

Compute the pH Average

After three or four days of saliva and urine readings, you want to take the average of all reading. Here is how you can determine what your pH readings mean.

pH level of 6.5 to 7.4 - You are at a **healthy level.** However, the higher number is better.

pH level of 6.0 to 6.5 – You may **not be feeling good and need to make some changes in your diet.**

pH level of 5.0 to 6.0 - You have **major health problems.**
pH level of 4.5 – 5.0 – You **have a terminal disease.**

You are considered to have an alkaline body, if your overall body pH liquids are 6.5 to 7.4. This is the pH level that you should strive for. Higher pH values of 7.5 to 8.5 and up are considered detrimental.

pH and Body Oxygen

Another important issue related to pH is the oxygen level. Tissue and cells have more oxygen available to them when your body pH is 7.4 as compared to when it is 6.4.

It has been found that the average American's tissue pH is between 5.5 and 6.0, an acid body. This indicates that they have a severe lack of oxygen in their cells and lymph liquid. Lack of oxygen in the body is known to create serious terminal diseases. It is oxygen that destroys all types of bacteria and pathogens that live inside your body and make you ill.

Those of you with acid bodies and that lack cell and lymph oxygen can correct your condition by learning what it takes to bring your body back to an alkaline level. This will give your body a chance to repair tissue and organs, provided, they have not been severely damaged.

9: How Minerals Burn Acid And Relieve Gout

Minerals

Moving your body more toward alkalinity is what will give you the best health. When you have gout problems, getting more minerals in your body is the first step. An alkaline body prevents your body from becoming ill and forming deadly diseases, like joint problems, organ degradation, body pain, skin eruptions, cancer, and system weaknesses. If you are already sick, then all the chemicals inside fruits and vegetables will help revive you to better health. This is provided that your tissue damage has not gone beyond repair.

Uric acid also has higher solubility in solutions of alkali hydroxides and their carbonates than in acidic media. So making your body more alkaline, is what you need to do to reduce or eliminate gout.

If your urine pH is less than 5.5, uric acid crystals precipitate and lead to stone formation. If the urine is neutral or alkaline, pH 7.0 to 7.4, uric acid remains in solution and does not precipitate. At 37°C and pH 6.6, the solubility of uric acid is 6 mg per 100 ml, whereas at pH 7.0, uric acid is almost three times more soluble and stable.

The minerals most important in changing and maintaining your body in an alkaline condition are sodium, potassium, solutions at concentrations of 16 mg per 100 ml. Other mineral such as chloride, calcium, phosphorus, magnesium, and sulfur are also critical in making your body alkaline.

Acid Binding

There are certain minerals that are called acid binding. And these are minerals, as mentioned earlier, are the most important ones for gout, sodium, potassium, chloride, calcium, phosphorus, magnesium, because they are acid binding.

What acid binding means is when you eat fruits with these minerals, your cells, after using them, create an alkaline ash. This ash will seek out acids in your body and bind with them to neutralize them. These captured acids are then routed out of your body through your urine, stools, and breathe.

Since acids in your body are toxic, your body has the priority of getting rid of them fast. If they are not removed, you form an acid body and these acids will damage tissue, cause pain, and disease.

So you can see the importance of getting a lot of alkaline minerals into your body. Without them, acids, which do not get bonded to alkaline minerals, would move back into body tissue and continue their body damage.

Keeping Healthy

One of the most important parts of health is keeping the lymph liquid around your cells clean and free of toxins. To do this you need to provide alkaline minerals to occupy the lymph liquid, and you need to remove the acids that accumulate in that liquid and in all parts of your body tissue. You can do this by detoxifying your body and providing alkaline minerals for your lymph liquid.

Body Detoxification

The highest priority of the body is to detoxify itself. One of the best ways to help your body detoxify is to provide minerals that bind with acids that are in the cells, tissues, organs, and muscles. What these alkaline acid binding minerals do is to pull out the toxins that are dispersed throughout your body.

By eating fruits and vegetables and their minerals, your body is constantly detoxifying itself. But when it is over loaded with acid toxins, from your lifestyle, a complete detox of your body becomes impossible, unless you do a three to seven day body cleanse.

Emotional Toxins

But there is another factor that creates acid in your body and that is emotions that are occur through life stresses, like work pressures, divorce, friendship problems, martial issues, and other similar problems. These emotional problems create acidic molecules that embed themselves into your tissues, just like food acids.

Body Organs

All body organs function to rid the body of acid waste or toxins. Lack of acid binding food causes deterioration of the function of these organs. Each organ has a specific function in the elimination and neutralization of acid wastes and it does this in conjunction with acid binding minerals.

Here is a list of fruits, vegetables, and other foods that have the highest alkaline minerals and the highest acid production. The percentage number next to these foods indicates the strength of the alkaline minerals or the acid minerals.

The closer to 100% the more effective these foods are as an acid reducing food. However, you should be eating all foods throughout the list not just the ones at the top of the list.

The percentage assigned to these fruits is based on fresh fruits and vegetables that are organic and not cooked canned or mixed with sugar. If they are cooked or otherwise processed in some fashion, this will slightly reduce their effectiveness as an acid binding. However, they will still be effective in some acid binding.

Acid Binding Fruits With Alkaline Minerals

In the list below are fruits and vegetables with alkaline minerals that create acid binding salts in your body, used to neutralize acid wastes. Foods above 50% in value are more acid binding, which means they will more trap or bind with acid wastes. Foods below 50% are more acid producing and are called alkaline binding, since they tie up or bind with alkaline minerals. This means a loss of alkaline minerals that you need to neutralize acids.

To create an alkaline body, you need to eat 80% acid binding food and 20% alkaline binding food. Work towards this end and you will slowly move your body from acid to alkaline.
Here is the list of foods to eat in the order of priority.

Fruits

Fruits at 100% Acid Binding – Best Fruits To Eat
Lemons, melons – any type, watermelon

Fruits at 93% Acid Binding – Great Fruits To Eat
Cantaloupes, dried dates, dried figs, limes, mango, papaya

Fruits at 87% Acid Binding – Still Great Fruits To Eat
Kiwis, passion Fruit, pineapples, raisins, umeboshi plums

Fruits at 80% Acid Binding – Eat These Fruits
Apricots, avocados, bananas, fresh dates, fresh figs, currants, gooseberries grapes, guavas, kumquats, nectarines, pears, persimmons, quince, berries, cactus

Fruits 73% Acid Binding – Still Fruits To Eat
Apples, oranges, peaches, pomegranate, raspberries, sour grapes, strawberries, carob

Fruits at 67% Acid Binding – Still Neutralizes Acids
Cherries, fresh coconut

Herbal Teas From Leaves at 73% to 86% acid binding Alfalfa, mint, sage, spearmint, raspberry strawberry comfrey

All Herbs and Spices at 67% to 73% Acid Binding

Fruits 40% to 47% - Eat less of these fruits Blueberries, cranberries, plums, prunes

All Juices from a juicer 100% Acid Binding

Vegetables

Here is the list of vegetables to eat for gout in order of priority. All of these vegetables will neutralize acid, since they contain minerals that are acid binding.

Vegetables at 93% Acid Binding – best vegetables to eat Kelp, Seaweed, Watercress, Asparagus

Vegetables at 80% Acid Binding – Still the best to eat Lettuce Leaf, Oyster plant, Pumpkin, Spinach, Squash, Peas, Carrots, Celery, Chard, Swiss, Dandelion greens

Vegetables at 73% Acid Binding – Great vegetables to eat Bamboo shoots, Beets, Broccoli, Cabbage, Cauliflower, Collards, Corn, sweet, Ginger (fresh), Mushrooms, Mustard greens, Onions, Pepper, Potatoes, Green, Lima, String, Potatoes

Vegetables at 67% Acid Binding – eat plenty of these Brussels sprouts, Cucumbers, Eggplant, Okra, Onions, Radishes, Tomatoes

Vegetable juices at 80% to 93% Acid Binding Parsley, wheat grass, carrot, celery, etc.

Soy Bean Products at 60% Acid Binding – limit your use of tofu since it is a genetically modified organism, GMO Dried beans, Soy cheese, Soy milk, Tempeh, Tofu

Other Foods For Gout

Here are some other misc. foods to eat that are acid binding. Starches at 80% Acid Binding

Nuts and Seeds at 60 % to 67% Acid Binding
Almonds, sesame seeds, Granola, Essene Bread, Chestnuts

Misc. foods at 60% Acid Binding

Horseradish, Amaranth, Millet, Quinoa, Dried beans, Soy cheese, Soy milk,

The following foods are alkaline binding, which means that they create acids that will bind with alkaline salts and remove them from your body. These foods when eaten in excess will create an acid body.

You should only eat around 20% of these foods in your diet, and the other 80% should come from fruits and vegetables or foods that are acid binding.

NOTE: The lower the alkaline binding percentage, the more that food is acid producing.

Oils

All oils are basically at 50% and are considered neutral. This includes almond, avocado, canola, coconut, corn castor, olive, soy, sunflower oil, etc.

Food That Creates Acid

Beans, starches, and nuts and seeds at 40% to 46% Alkaline Binding and create body acid.

Aduki, Black, Broadbean, Garbanzo, Mung, Pinto, Barley, Corn Meal, Lentils, Brans, Cashews, Coconut (dried), Pecans, Brans, Millet, Filberts, Walnuts, Pumpkin, Sunflower
Starches at 26 to 33 % Alkaline Binding or highly acidic
Brown Rice, Buckwheat, Oats, Spelt, Wheat Whole, Peanuts, corn, rye

Rice at 20% Alkaline Binding and highly acidic
White rice

Sugar at 13% Alkaline Binding, highly acidic
White beet or cane sugar
Meat and Fish

Meat at 26% alkaline binding highly acidic
Fish With fins and scales, Shellfish - shrimp, scallops, crab lobster, oyster

Meat at 20% Alkaline Binding, highly acidic
Chicken, turkey, rabbit

Meat at 13% Alkaline Binding, highly acidic
Beef, goat, pork, lamb

Misc. Products at 13% to 26% Alkaline Binding highly acidic
Liquor, wine, beer, coffee, black tea, caffeine drinks

10: Body Cycles That Stop Gout

Body cycles are time periods where your body is doing certain functions in your body. It does this automatically, as if it was on a timer. Knowing what these functions are, will help you get relief from your disease and even eliminate it. You should use these cycles outline below every day.

Here are the 3 natural body cycles:

Cycle 1 time period: 4 a.m. to noon

This cycle is the time where your body is eliminating toxins, acids, wastes, and derby through urine, bowel movements, and other secretions. Most people interfere with this cycle, since they are unaware of it, causing constipation, increase weight and various detrimental illnesses.

Cycle 2 time period: noon to 8 p.m.

This is the time when your body should be taking in food and digesting it. By eating the right kind of food, you help your digestive process in your stomach and small intestine. This is your first and second meal of the day – lunch and dinner.

Cycle 3 time period: 8 p.m. to 4 a.m.

This is the time your body is absorbing and using food you have eaten from noon to 8 p.m. Various organs are detoxifying and producing waste and moving it into your kidneys and colon. When you wake up, this is the waste you should be getting rid during body cycle one.

The First Body Cycle

During the elimination cycle, 4 a.m. to noon, eat and drink only fruits and their juices or vegetable juices. For breakfast, eat a bowl of fruits or have a fruit smoothie made with apple juice, banana, and fruits in season.

Before noontime, eat fruits as snacks. Forty-five minutes before noon, eat your last fruit. You can eat and drink all the fruits and juices you want up to noontime.

Fruits contain the right balance of nutrients, with about 70% distilled water. Eat them without cooking them. They are easy to digest and absorb and do not stress your colon. They activate peristaltic action in your colon and help you have a bowel movement.

Use the Acid Binding fruits listed in the previous chapter. Here are some more fruits to eat:

Apples

Apricots

Avocados

Bananas

Blueberries

Boysenberries

Cantaloupes

Cherries

Figs and dates

Grapes

Grapes

Lemons

Nectarines

Oranges

Papayas

Peaches

Pears

Persimmons

Plums

Prunes

Raspberries

Strawberries

Watermelons

Eat all melons together and not with other fruit, and wait 1/2 hour before eating other fruit. Melons require specific enzymes to be digested in your stomach, so other fruits eaten with melons will just sit in your stomach, waiting to be digested. This will cause you gas and an acid stomach.

By eating fruits during body cycle 1, you are assisting your body's elimination cycle. Fruits and juices help your body to urinate, or have a bowel movement. They help you eliminate toxins and acids from your body and blood. It is these toxins and acids that make you, overweight, constipated, and sick.

Eating solid food for breakfast – eggs potatoes, rice, meat, cereal, milk, and so on, the typical breakfast, interferes with your body's elimination cycle and eventually leads to sickness and excess weight.

It takes over 3 hours to digest heavy and solid food. The food you should be eating in the morning should digest quickly. This helps you to activate peristaltic colon action to create a bowel movement and to continue your body's detoxification and elimination process.

Heavy food slows down the elimination of toxins from your body, and this causes fecal matter and toxins to remain in your colon longer than necessary. These toxins then get stored in your body, as fat and acids.

It takes 1 to 1 1/2 hour or so to digest fruits and fruit juices. Because of this, they help to cleanse your body of waste during the time from 4am to noontime.

So if you are not already having fruits and fruits and vegetables juices for breakfast and snacks, start slowing changing your eating habits. This will help you detoxify your body daily, lose weight, create an alkaline body, and eliminate your gout.

The Second Natural Body Cycle

Here is the second body cycle, and it occurs from noon to 8 p.m.

This is the time when your body should be taking in food and digesting it. During this period, it is time to eat solid food. What you eat has to be in alignment with what your stomach can do.

Here's how your stomach works. In generally it can only digest one solid food at a time.

A solid food is one that does not contain 70% water, like fruits and vegetables do, and whose water has been eliminated by heat or other food processes, in other words, cooked.

Your stomach can only work on one solid food at a time, so your lunch and dinner should only have one solid food. A lunch can consist of chicken and a green salad, fish and a green salad, tuna and a green salad, shrimp and a green salad, beef and a green salad.

Mixing a protein meal with carbohydrates is giving the stomach two solid foods at the same time, which require different concentrations of digestive juices.

When you eat any animal protein, avoid eating it with non-starchy vegetables - artichokes, yams, sweet potatoes, carrots, oats, peas, potatoes, rice, wheat, winter squash and corn. These vegetables break down into sugars that coat your protein food and this causes a chemical process called glycation, which creates inflammation and lowers your immunity. In addition, this combination of protein and starches are difficult to digest and disrupt your second body cycle.

When you eat animal protein, eat it with broccoli, cabbage, cauliflower, celery, cucumber, garlic, green beans, leafy greens onions, garlic, wakame, dulse, and zucchini.

Giving the stomach more than it can handle interrupts the elimination cycle 1 and reduces the energy that you need, during this morning cycle.

Here's how you can help your body's cycle 2 to be more effective.

Eat only one solid food with vegetables during lunch or dinner. Lunch can be one meat or seafood with a fresh vegetable salad that is non-starchy.

Or you can eat only brown or red rice or other grains, with both starchy and non-starchy vegetables, with no meat.

Limit the amount of water you drink during meals. Excess water will dilute your digestive acids and slow down the digestion of your food.

Avoid drinking sodas, tea or other drinks, during your meals. If you need to clear your dry throat, use room-temperature water. Cold liquids will slow down your digestive processes.

Eating meals with more than one solid food, such as meat and potatoes, chicken and rice, fish and rice, chicken and noodles, eggs and toast, cheese and bread, will diminish the energy you need during the elimination cycle.

It is permissible to eat beef and chicken at the same time but not chicken and eggs or beef and nuts or chicken and beans. Eat the same type of protein at the same time, but do not mix different proteins.

It's ok to eat different types of carbohydrates at the same time, with a salad, but not with protein, since carbohydrates digest easier than protein.

Eating a variety of food at the same time leads to undigested food. Food that is partially undigested becomes acidic, which affects the health of your colon and causes gout. When these acids are absorbed into your body, they are converted into fat and stored as toxins your body.

Eating the right combination of foods at meal time helps you to preserve your energy for the elimination cycle. In addition, it prevents you from creating spoiled food in your stomach that is converted to acid waste. It is this acid waste that results in illness and fat. This is the reason most people, as they age, come down with various illnesses that terminate their lives early or gain excessive weight.

The Third Body Cycle

The third body cycle is the assimilation cycle and is from 8 pm to 4 am. This is the time the food you have eaten during the day is assimilated, absorbed and distributed throughout your body through your blood. It is the time where digested food moves into the colon as chime or fecal matter and is stored there for elimination. And, you should be eliminating this chime or fecal matter, when you wake up or during the morning to noon.

Food eaten during the second cycle, noon to 8 p.m. and that were combined and eaten properly will digest within 3 to 4 hours. But, food not combined properly, a meal consisting of protein and carbohydrates will take up to 8 hours to pass through your stomach. During this time, your food will putrefy and ferment and become acidic. Under these conditions, you will not get many nutrients from that meal.

So, eat your last meal by 6-7 pm, so that your food digests in your stomach, by the time you go to bed. After three hours later, your food will have moved into your small intestine, where it is ready for assimilation.

When you go to bed 3 hours after your last meal, the next 6 hours, until 4am, your body will be absorbing the food you have eaten the previous day and moving waste into your colon and collecting urine in your bladder.

Gout Diet

11: Colon-Blood Cleanse That Reduces Gout Pain

One of the first things you need to do to get started on getting a healthier colon is to do a two to three day colon and blood cleanse. This is an important step because you want to remove toxins and mucus from your intestinal tract – stomach, small intestine, colon, and many other body organs. In this three day cleanse you will also remove toxins from within your cells and lymph liquid.

This cleanse will pullout many of the acids, acid wastes, and toxins you have floating around in your body. This makes your body more alkaline.

This cleanse will clean out your blood and neutralize many of the acids in your body that are causing you harm. The cleanse will also pull out excess body water and reduce any edema that you might have. This will happen because this cleanse promotes urination and bowel movements.

Constipation

Part of this cleanse is to help you have regular bowel movements. If you do not have one to two bowel movements per day, your body will become toxic. Some toxins are often converted to fat. Keeping regular helps to keep your body clear of toxins and helps to keep your weight down.

To help you clear out your colon, there are two ways to do this, in this cleanse. You can take Oxypowder during your three day cleanse or you can drink prune juice in a special way.

In this cleanse, you will only be drinking vegetable juices, fruit juices and eating some fruits for three days. Doing a juice cleanse can give you some side effects, where you feel nauseated or slightly sick.

Not everyone will get these effects. If you feel sick, this is a sign that you are stirring up toxins in your stomach and elsewhere in your body, and as you get rid of these toxins, you will begin to feel better.

In her extensive book, Cooking For Healthy Healing, 1991, Linda Rector-page, N.D., Ph.D., talks about what a fast does,

"Fasting works by self-digestion. During a cleanse, the body in its infinite wisdom, will decompose and burn only the substances and tissue that are damaged, diseased, or unneeded, such as abscesses, tumors, excess fat deposits, and congestive wastes. Even a relatively short fast can accelerate elimination from the kidneys, liver, lungs and skin, often causing dramatic changes as masses of accumulated waste is expelled. Live foods and juices can literally pick up dead matter from the body and carry it away."

So, here's what you need to do to get started.

The Day Before The Cleanse

Buy the following juices for this cleanse a few days before or the day before your cleanse.

Organic apple juice – one gallon

Organic apples – 3 for one day, 10 apples for three days

Organic prune juice – 1/2 gallon

Organic Cherry juice – 1/2 gallon

Carrots for your juicer or carrot juice – one quart

The day before the fast, eat a large salad and two apples at dinner time. This will give you plenty of fiber to scrub the walls of your colon as you move fecal matter out of your colon the following day.

Cleansing the Colon

If you chose to use Oxy-Powder, then here is where you can buy it on the Internet: <u>Get Oxy-Powder</u>

The night before you start your cleanse, take four Oxy-Powder capsules, just before bedtime.

Now, Oxy-Powder is not a laxative, so it is not addictive. What these capsules do is supply oxygen to your colon, which dissolves the hard fecal matter that has built up over time and has not wanted to come out.

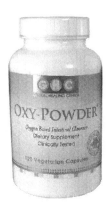

Because this bottle of Oxy-Powder has 125 capsules, you can take 4 to 5 capsules during your 3 day cleanse.

Oxy-Powder causes your stools to become watery, since it is dissolving the hard matter in your colon. Don't be concerned that you have diarrhea like symptoms. Also this three day cleanse will also cause you to have watery stools, since you are on a diet of juices and vegetables.

If you chose to use prune juice to clear out your colon, this procedure will be described below.

First day of colon cleanse

Do this cleanse on a Saturday, Sunday or any other day that you don't have to go anywhere. You may be going to the bathroom all day, and at times you need to be there quick. But, you can do this cleanse even during a workday.

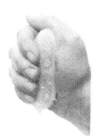 This first morning, you will have a bowel movement, when you wake up, because of the Oxy-Powder. After that, go do your lemon drink.

Lemon Juice Drink - Every morning when you first get up, drink a glass of slightly warm water, with the juice of 1/2 lemon. This will remove mucus from your intestinal tract and detoxify your colon.

Prune Juice Colon Cleanse

If you decided to use prune juice to clean out your colon, instead of Oxy-Powder, then here is what you need to do.

But you can also do prune juice, if you have done the Oxy-powder, since prune juice is filled with minerals and nutrients that will cleanse your body.

About 1/2 hour after your lemon drink, take 8 oz. of prune juice.

- 5 to 10 minutes later, drink another 8 oz. of prune juice

- 5 to 10 minutes later, again drink another 8 oz. of prune juice

- wait 20 minutes, then drink 8 oz. of apple juice

- wait 30 minutes, then drink another 8 oz. of apple juice

If you haven't sped to the bathroom yet, you will in a little while.

Now drink 8 oz. of apple juice, every hour until the end of the day. You can stop drinking apple juice around 5pm. You can use different fruit juices or vegetable juices in place of apple juice, but, just make sure you drink plenty apple juice.

During the day, you can eat 1 or 2 apple in the morning and 1 or 2 in the evening.

Second Day Of The Colon Cleanse

During the second day, you can drink different kinds of juices and eat 2-6 apples. You can drink any kind of juice be it fruit or vegetable. A combination of juice and vegetable juice is good. You can now eat other fruits, such as watermelon, melon, oranges, and strawberries.

Third Day Of The Colon Cleanse

The third day is like the second day where you can drink different kinds of juice and eat 2-6 apples or other fruits.

On this day, you can eat other fruits, like mango, watermelon, cantaloupe, and pineapple. At the end of this day, you can eat a salad with a variety of vegetables.

Fourth Day Start Of Colon Cleanse

If you are using Oxypowder, take 3-4 capsule before bedtime and 2-4 capsule in the morning, during each day of your cleanse.

You can continue to use Oxypowder at 2 -3 capsules every night for the rest of the month.

12: Exercises That Strengthen Your Immune System

Caution: If you have not exercised for a while, take this program slowly and work into it. If you feel some concern about exercising and your health, made sure you see your doctor.

You want to include some exercise for gout. But you need to work into it slowly, especially if you have gout in your feet or legs. In this case, you want to wait until your gout is gone.

Once you have eliminated gout, you need to exercise to strengthen your various joints and muscles. Start with walking and increase your range slightly every week.

Once you feel better, here is a more strenuous exercise program that you can work into. This program that is one of the best for maintaining your health, and you don't have to do more than 15 minutes, but start with 5 minutes and do your exercises slowly and work up on speed and movement.

Get Started

So let's get started with the exercises you need to do. You will be doing these exercises in a different way than you are used to. Most exercise gurus tell you that you need aerobics to strengthen your hearts. Exercise studies have shown that this is not the way to strengthen your heart; in fact it does the opposite. When you go to the gym for and do repetitive exercises for over 20 minutes you are not strengthening your heart.

In his e-book called Pace, Dr. Al Sears outlines a new way of exercising to strengthen your cardiovascular system. He says that, "During twenty years of working with extremely fit athletes, patients with diseased or injured hearts and average people in between, one thing is apparent: Doing what we have come to accept as 'cardio' exercise is a waste of your time and effort.

It doesn't build what your heart really needs. It doesn't increase your heart's ability to respond to the real demands. In fact, for all your effort, you only reduce your ability to handle suddenly demanding events that may come your way – the last thing you want."

During the short, fast exercises from 2 to 15 minutes, you are burning calories supplied by:

The first couple of minutes the energy comes from your ATP – cell energy.

After 2 minutes, the energy comes from the carbohydrates stored in your muscle tissue.

After 15-20 minutes, the energy starts to come from stored fat. When you exercise at a moderate rate you are burning 40% carbohydrates and 55% fat. When your exercise at a high intensity, you are burning 95% carbohydrates and 3% fat. You want to exercise in a way and for time duration where you are burning carbohydrates and very little fat.

Anaerobic Exercise

The way you will exercise is to exercise for short duration at high intensity. This is called anaerobic exercise. To do anaerobic exercise you exercise at a pace you can't sustain for more than a short time. You will be breathing hard and are asking your lungs for more oxygen than they can give you.

Because of this, your lungs need to expand to get more oxygen. You are now building your lungs for greater capacity. You are now burning more carbohydrates than fat. And, in the time between exercising your fat is burned since your body determines it is not necessary to keep fat for energy since carbohydrates are what is really needed.

So what are the benefits of doing these anaerobic exercises?

- Reverse heart disease
- Lower cholesterol
- Reduce high blood pressure
- Increase oxygen in your blood
- Increase lung capacity
- Strengthen your immune system
- Reverse changes of aging

All of these benefits create cleaner arteries and more blood flow to the kidneys to remove uric acids.

Exercising

As you do Pace exercises, you will change your routine each time you exercise. Instead of exercising longer, you will increase the exercise intensity and the resistive element of exercising.

To start this exercise program, start with a 10 minute workout. You can do your exercise on a stair-stepper, stationary bike, treadmill, run, swim, or ride your bike.

Doctor Check

You will want to check with your doctor, if you:

- Have had not a medical checkup during the past two years

- Are over 50

- Are 26 lbs or over

- Have heart pains, chest pains, or rapid heart palpitations after you exercise

- Are taking heart medication or have a pace maker

- Have angina, heart murmur or any type of heart disease

- Have a relative who died of a heart attack before the age of 60

- Have a hard time breathing and have any type of respiratory disease – asthma, emphysema.

Monitoring Your Heart Rate

To check your progress in your exercise program, you need to check your:

- Resting heart rate
- Maximum heart rate for your age
- Maximum heart rate during exercise
- Recovery heart rate

Resting Heart Rate

Your resting heart rate is the rate before you exercise. The lower your resting heart rate is the healthier you are, unless you heart problems. A normal rate is 60 to 100 pulses per minute. If you are really in good shape, then your pulse will be 40 – 60 per minute.

To determine your resting heart rate get a second timer and count the number of pulses you have in 10 seconds. Then multiple this number by 6 to get your pulse rate per minute.
To get a more accurate reading of your pulse rate do your 10 second reading 3 time and get an average of these readings.

Maximum Heart Rate for Your Age

The maximum heart rate for your age is that heart rate that you should strive for during your exercise to get the best benefit of your exercise. You calculate this rate by subtracting your age from 220. During your exercise, you want to achieve 60- 80 % of your maximum heart rate for your age. Here is a sample chart you can use to see different heart rates for your heart:

Age	Max Pulse 220-age	60% of max pulse	80% of max pulse
35	185	111	148
40	180	108	144
45	175	105	140
50	170	102	136
55	165	99	132
60	160	96	128
65	155	93	124
70	150	90	120

Based on your physical condition, use these numbers as guide lines.

Maximum Heart Rate During Exercise

The maximum heart rate is the highest rate your pulse achieved during your exercise. Use the chart about to evaluate where you are with respect to the heart rate for your age. During exercise if your heart rate is on the lower end of the heart rate for your age, you will want to exercise harder to get your heart rate up. If you are really out of shape, then take it easy and work up to the 60% and eventually to the 80% heart rate as you improve your stamina.

You can measure your exercise heart rate the same way you calculate your resting heart rate.

Recovery Heart Rate

Your heart recovery rate is the time it takes for your maximum heart rate to recover to your resting heart rate. As you exercise more, the less time will be required for you to achieve your heart recovery rate. When you exercise for your chosen time, clock your recovery rate, since a change in this rate indicates you are improving in your health. You will see change in this rate in one month. Do not do your next exercise until you reach your resting heart rate. So you will be cycling from resting rate –exercise rate – resting rate – exercise rate – resting rate. Do five to ten of these cycles as an exercise routine.

Caution: See your doctor, before you start an exercise program or if the following conditions occur:

Your heart rate, after maximum exercise, does not come

- down within a few minutes
- You feel dizzy or faint
- You have chest pains or are short of breath
- You have rapid heartbeat or irregular heartbeat

This exercise program is the basic outline of Dr. Sears' PACE program. His e-book takes off to higher levels of exercise methods, so if you want to see his full program you can buy his e-book called **Pace: The 12-Minute Fitness Revolution**

13: A Program to Stop and Eliminate Gout

I provided you with a lot of information on various aspects of gout. This gives you a chance to see what action you need to take, to get rid of it and to cure it.

I have given many things to do and natural remedies and supplements to take. The reason for this is so that you can first find those remedies that you might already have in your kitchen or refrigerator. If you have these foods or remedies, you can get started right away, getting some pain relief.

One of the secrets of curing gout is using the idea that gout is an acid-alkaline imbalance. So, what this means is that you need to stop eating and doing those things that are causing this imbalance in your body.

What this imbalance means is that you have too much acid in your body, which causes uric acid to precipitate out of your blood and create crystals that end up in your joints.

Here is an outline of how to get started.

- Start drinking more water. You want to urinate more to reduce the amount of uric acid you have in your body.

- You want to drink fruit and vegetable juices that give you more acid binding minerals, like watermelon, various juices, fruits, and herbal remedy teas. Use more fruits and vegetables that give you 80 to 100% acid binding results.

- You need to get rid of the excess acid in your body. So you need to do the **3 day colon and blood cleanse.**

This cleanse will pull out your excess body acids in your blood, lymph liquid, and around and inside your cells.

Make some changes in the way you eat.

- Look at the list of foods to avoid. You don't have to be perfect here, just start minimizing their use.

- Then look at the food to eat more of and start adding them into your diet.

Start using some of the natural remedies. Look over the list and choose a couple of them.

- Pick a couple of them and use them for a week to see if you see a difference in your condition. Keep trying different ones, until you find one that works for you. You can do short time test, to see if any of remedies give you quick relief.

Now take a look at the various supplements that are good for gout.

- Use kelp and celery seeds to help reduce body acid

- Use digestive enzymes to help you digestion your food better, so that you don't create a lot of stomach acid waste

Gets pH paper so you can see how acidic you are.

- Use pH paper for a few months, so you can monitor your condition and progress.

Creating a more alkaline body will go a long way in improving your overall health.

Read over the section on Burning Acid. There is a chart there that tells you the best fruits and vegetables to eat to create an acid body. You need to concentration on this produce.

For example, here are the top fruits to eat:

- Fruits at 100% Acid Binding – Best fruits To Eat Lemons, melons – any type, watermelon

- Fruits at 93% Acid Binding – great fruits To Eat Cantaloupes, dried dates, dried figs, limes, mango, papaya

But don't neglect the other fruits.

For the top vegetables to eat here is the start:

- Vegetables at 93% Acid Binding – best vegetables to eat Kelp, Seaweed, Watercress, Asparagus

Vegetables at 80% Acid Binding – Still the best to eat Lettuce Leaf, Oyster plant, Pumpkin, Spinach, Squash, Peas, Carrots, Celery, Chard, Swiss, Dandelion greens

There is still one more important thing to do:

- Change the way and what you eat for breakfast.

In the Body Cycle chapter, I go over how to eat breakfast.

- Use the best fruits or vegetables for breakfast.

This will help you to detoxify your body and eliminate and neutralize acids daily. This one of the best health practices you can do for your body.

After your gout is gone, start an exercising program, but start out slowly, if you have not been exercising, work up to higher levels, using the Pace Program.

There you have it, a comprehensive health program that is super for getting rid of gout and giving you better overall health.

Use these principles and you will gain new health and happiness.

14: Author And Resources

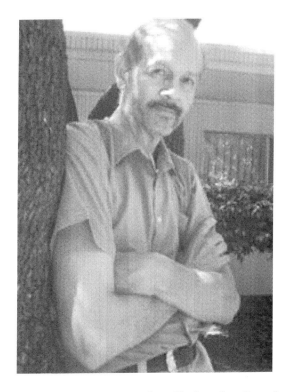

Get one of my best kindle books *free* below:

http://www.natural-remedies-thatwork.com

Rudy Silva is a natural consultant nutritionist educated in the United States in Nutrition and Physics. He is a graduate from the San Jose State University in California. He is author of 45 other books on natural remedies. He has authored a newsletter in natural remedies for over 4 years.

Resource page

Here are some of the other kindle e-books about natural remedies that have been written by this author. You can see the entire list at:

http://tinyurl.com/b2f7wd3

Constipation Remedies
Best Constipated Women Natural Cures

Essential Fatty Acids
Taking The Mystery Out Of Essential Fatty acids
Amazing Fish Oil Benefits Revealed

Nutrition Remedies
Fast Healing Juice Nutrition Therapy: Nutrition Tips 3
Magnesium Nutrition Revealed
Potassium Health Secrets Revealed

Stomach Remedies
Acid Reflux: Fast and Easy Cures For Acid Reflux
Asthma Treatment Cures With Remedies
How To Do Natural Colon Cleansing

Misc. Remedies
Effective Natural Hemorrhoids Treatment
Iron Deficiency Anemia
Best Varicose Vein Treatments?

Men's Health
Best Impotence Health Diet

Weight loss

Ten (10) Day Quick Success Weight Loss Program

To see all of the kindle books written by this author, go to the Authors Profile Page or this URL:

http://tinyurl.com/b2f7wd3

If you need support or want to promote any of his e-books, please contact him at rss41@yahoo.com and expect a reply within 24 hours.

Give A Review

And, don't forget to give a review for this e-book at Amazon. It's not hard to give a review. It can be only a sentence or two. You don't have to leave a long review. A short review helps other people decide if they want to buy a book. So give a short review and give your thoughts to help other people and to help the author improve his book.

To you, for creating better health and more happiness,

Rudy S Silva

Made in the USA
Lexington, KY
03 November 2015